Using
Interactive Art
as a
Therapeutic Tool

Karen E. Erdman, RN, BSN, MEd

WestBow Press books may be ordered through booksellers or by contacting:

WestBow Press
A Division of Thomas Nelson & Zondervan
1663 Liberty Drive
Bloomington, IN 47403
www.westbowpress.com
844-714-3454

Scripture quotations marked NIV are taken from the Holy Bible, New International Version®, NIV®. Copyright © 1973, 1978, 1984 by Biblica, Inc.™ Used by permission of Zondervan. All rights reserved worldwide.

Scripture quotations marked KJV are taken from the Holy Bible, King James Version.

ISBN: 979-8-3850-2563-3 (sc)
ISBN: 979-8-3850-2564-0 (hc)
ISBN: 979-8-3850-2565-7 (e)

Library of Congress Control Number: 2024909949

Print information available on the last page.

WestBow Press rev. date: 02/12/2025

Contents

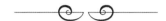

List of Graphics v

Acknowledgments vii

Chapter 1   Where Did That Come From?.. 1

Chapter 2   The Purpose of Using Interactive Art as a Therapeutic Tool...................... 3

Chapter 3   Rooms in My Heart—Sadie's Story.. 7

Chapter 4   Suggested Ways to Use Rooms in My Heart Print..................................... 11

Chapter 5   Rooms in My Heart—Christian Perspective and Forgiveness............................. 13

Chapter 6   Rooms in My Heart—Partners and Family 15

Chapter 7   Other Prints as Therapeutic Tools 17

Chapter 8   Testimony 39

Chapter 9   Message to the Reader 43

Chapter 10   The Amen Chapter... 45

Suggested Reading... 47

References 49

Scripture References.. 50

Response/Evaluation Sheet.. 51

Blank Note Pages 53

List of Graphics

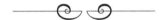

Image Title Sheet 1, *Rooms in My Heart* print

Image Title Sheet 2, *Wisdom Tree* print

Image Title Sheet 3, *Tread On* print

Image Title Sheet 4, *Fallen Leaves* print

Image Title Sheet 5, *Salvation* print

Image Title Sheet 6, *Party Balloons* (15) print

Image Title Sheet 7, *Party Balloons* (9) print

Image Title Sheet 8, *Label Me Bright* print

Image Title Sheet 9, *Camouflage* print

Acknowledgments

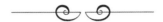

Heavenly Father, thank you for allowing this clay vessel to carry Your thoughts and designs to others so that they may be released from chains. If there is any good to be found and shared through using this workbook, to God goes the glory.

Lamar, you are not only my partner in life and my emotional support, but you are a total whiz with all my IT challenges. Thank you, my love. I appreciate beyond words that you have always said, "Whatever you feel led to do, do it."

Deborah, I am sure you never intended to be an integral part of this book's existence, but you are. You have been woven into the very fabric of it. Your prayers and presence are not by luck, not by chance, and not by accident. God knew exactly which of your many talents I would need to tap into. Thank you for your kind and gracious generosity!

Thank you so very much, Deb A., Karen, Robin, Bob, Lena, Janet, Jimmy, and so many other people for your prayers, encouragement, input, and support. You are irreplaceable and valued more than you will ever know!

Recovery is a process. It takes time.
It takes patience. It takes everything you've got.
—unknown

CHAPTER 1

Where Did That Come From?

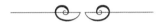

A year and a half after being widowed, I was about to commit my life—and the lives of my two young sons—to a second marriage. I was blessed but more than a little nervous. Even though my second husband was a wonderful man, I was certainly filled with my share of trepidation and concern regarding the relationship. I was unsettled mainly because I could not see into the future. I was not 100 percent sure that my marriage would not have a negative effect on my sons. I never saw or felt any dangerous warning signs before our wedding; it was the future that I was uncertain about. Nonetheless, I moved forward, banking on the marriage affecting my sons in a positive way. I was trusting God.

I am thrilled to say that was forty-four years ago. For those forty-four years, my husband has thought of those boys as his, and our sons truly know him as Dad in their hearts. Obviously, they know he is not their biological father, but he certainly is their dad.

Shortly after my second husband and I were married, one of my dear friends said, "Oh, I just hate you, Karen Erdman!"

This took me by surprise, in that she was one of my closest friends. I replied, "Ooookaaaay," but I thought, *Where did* that *come from?* I then asked her, "May I ask the reason why?"

My buddy said, "You have been married to two of the most wonderful men on the face of this earth, and I haven't found one yet!"

I couldn't help but smile and reply, "OK, yep, you can hate me for that reason."

She turned to me and said, "All kidding aside, can I ask you a serious question? You loved two men. How do you keep them separated in your head? How do you love them both without mixing them up or comparing them?"

I had to think for a minute. How could I explain what I felt and had experienced? Then I saw in my mind a picture of a heart filled with many, many "rooms," or spaces. I told her, "It is like having two children, two parents, or several friends for whom you have deep feelings." I pointed out to her that she would not mix up her love for her two brothers. She had different memories that she shared with each sibling, and each had his own personality. Their personalities, coupled with the memories she shared with each brother, made them each a unique individual. She could love them equally yet differently for who they were.

I told her, "My feelings for my two husbands were like that. I could appreciate each one for being an individual with his own personality. Their personalities and all the memories I shared with each spouse made them distinct. I loved them both but for different reasons."

I explained to her that it was as if we create a separate "room" in our hearts for each person we know. Memories and feelings are kept in the specific room that each person "occupies." Both positive and painful memories are housed there. No one else can enter, alter, or add to the memories or change our feelings that are stored there except us—and, of course, the "occupant" of each room.

"I get it!" she said. She understood that the owner of the heart could spend time with each occupant of a room, adding to the memories and feelings that were held there.

If the occupant of a room is removed from our lives due to certain circumstances, such as death, as my first husband was, then the door of that room is shut. No new memories can be added to the room. But the owner of the heart can still enter the room, spend time in the memories, and feel the love he or she has for that person. The memories, love, and emotions remain.

That was the genesis of my artwork *Rooms in My Heart* (*RIMH*). (The reader should understand that the *Rooms in My Heart* print has much more meaning, which I will explain in later chapters.)

Sometimes, however, the memories we hold are not good ones. Some of the memories that are locked inside us are painful, harmful, and beyond unpleasant. Sometimes those memories are detrimental or destructive to the person whose heart holds them. Those memories can cause a person to be eaten alive from the inside out, as if they're a cancer in the person's life.

And so, there is more to be shared.

CHAPTER 2

The Purpose of Using Interactive Art as a Therapeutic Tool

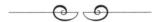

The main purpose of the interactive art (IA) prints is as a *tool* to assist counselors, psychologists, psychiatrists, clergy, therapists, and individuals in the emotional and mental healing process. The prints allow clients or individuals to move toward healthier thoughts, emotional relief, and positive emotional support. Simply, IA prints are instruments designed to aid in changing the mindset of a hurting client, family, group, or individual after experiencing an emotional tragedy.

A carpenter cannot work unless he or she has tools to do the job. A contractor needs hammers, saws, drills, and ladders to complete each task. Such is the case with pastors, counselors, and therapists, who also need instruments to help complete their jobs of conveying positive directions and communication to those who are hurting and dealing with major problems in their lives.

In the medical field, a doctor may prescribe more than one treatment for a patient. When applicable, it makes sense to introduce more than one method of counseling if the client responds positively to the techniques. Also, using tools in a specific manner to which the individual responds best can be the key needed to unlock and release painful memories.

Presenting clients with books, reading material, written lessons, and group classwork or homework may not address their deepest needs. They may not be able to identify with what they are reading or assimilate the text into their own situations. Many clients are simply not readers due to the inability to use the thought processes it takes to read through information, especially when dealing with emotional trauma or upset. Even if the book or material given to them is outstanding, they simply may not be able to focus on the written word and utilize the complex thinking areas of their brains.

One personal example that comes to my mind is the time I had major surgery. Prior to the surgery, I had great expectations of reading mystery novels, doing some sketching, and even spending time painting during this perceived mini-vacation. None of that happened! My body was traumatized, and my mind followed suit. I was unable to focus my attention on anything other than healing and the medical apparatus that was attached to me. My brain kept saying, *What in the blue blazes has just happened?* I was astonished at how much control my wounded body had on my mind, causing a total lack of focus and creativity. Yes, I eventually healed. Along with that healing, my normal level of concentration returned when I was reading, drawing, painting, or using more complex thinking skills.

Clients—all humans, for that matter—normally fall into one or more of four categories of learning modes that open cognitive understanding and retention of information. The categories are visual, auditory, read/write, and kinesthetic. The acronym VARK has been attached to these learning sensory modalities, as presented in a study performed by Neil D. Fleming and Coleen E. Mills (1992). These four approaches loosely identify styles and preferences of integrating information into our minds. Interactive art is a tool that utilizes all four of these methods of learning styles and offers the potential of meeting individual learning needs. Hopefully, this will present an opening to assist the counselor in reaching the client's goals of healing through learning to change a painful mindset.

Although there is a mountain of existing literature and opinions regarding learning styles, the actual research is comparably scarce. Without causing any further controversy, let us at least agree that we are all individuals who have differing needs, strengths, weaknesses, and learning methods. It is most widely accepted in the educational arena that there are indeed four basic methods of learning styles, which can be mashed together, pulled apart, and utilized as uniquely as each person's individual brain has designed.

The V in VARK represents visual learning. Studies have been performed on those people who would clearly identify as visual learners, and the results vary greatly. Sixty-five to 85 to 100 percent of the subjects state they strongly identify as visual learners.

> Research confirms video improves learning results. In addition, 90 percent of information transmitted to the brain is visual, and visuals are processed 60,000 times faster in the brain than text. This indicates visual education aids like video can improve learning styles and increase the rate at which we retain information.
>
> My company, Kaltura, recently published the inaugural State of Video in Education report in which more than 500 educational professionals from across 300 institutions unanimously agreed that video has the potential to create a real impact on education.
>
> Forrester Research estimates *one minute* of online video equates to approximately 1.8 million written words. In addition, *90 percent* of information transmitted to the brain is visual, and visuals are processed 60,000 times faster in the brain than text. (Tsur 2014)

Have you ever read a young children's book that did not have pictures? Probably not. I know I have not. That is because young children look at the pictures as someone reads the story to them. Children can see and hear the story come to life. As children grow older and learn to read for themselves, they need fewer pictures. The old saying, "A picture is worth a thousand words," holds true for many children and adults alike. Interactive art is a tangible tool, a visual instrument, that can be useful in aiding in the fight against invisible emotional distresses.

These facts certainly suggest that the use of visuals would benefit the person who is trying to grasp a concept or retain or even change an idea. In the classroom, videos, graphs, charts, maps, and tables are among the visuals that educators use to help students learn and retain information.

The A in VARK indicates auditory learning. Obviously, it's necessary to talk things through with the client during a therapeutic session. If clients are auditory learners, they may engage quicker when they are presented with an auditory interaction via discussion with a counselor. Verbalization is personal and affords the counselor the opportunity to observe reactions, gather information, and listen as clients share their thoughts. Clearly, talking with the therapist is a powerful tool in healing. During therapeutic sessions, the interactive art prints are used not only as a means of verbal communication between client and therapist, but these prints also can be used so that the client can avoid making uncomfortable direct eye contact with the therapist. This may allow clients to express themselves without feeling self-conscious.

The third area of learning in the VARK line-up is R, which stands for reading and writing. This is precisely what the interactive art prints were designed for—writing on them! The attention to and importance of this art is *not* the art itself. The main purpose of the art is to hold what is *written on it* by the client. The art was created not only as a focus for what is written on it but how it can be used to release emotional and mental distress. Many people love to journal; keep logs, blogs, and diaries; make notes; or send written greetings—the list goes on. A therapist may encourage clients to use journaling for therapeutic reasons.

In the same way, an interactive art print is the keeper of memories, both good and bad. The goal is for the client to purge and heal from those unhealthy memories.

In the next chapters I will present suggestions for therapists and clients to use the prints and hopefully purge those painful memories.

Last of all, some receive information and guidance quicker and easier because they are kinesthetic learners. Kinesthetic knowledge is the last method of absorbing information and initiating change in VARK. This technique of learning reaches those who thrive on being involved. An action is important to them and allows concepts to sink deeper into their thoughts. These are hands-on learners. The interactive art prints serve as a kinesthetic tool when clients write on the print and actively participate in their therapy.

As a postsecondary adult instructor, I used every tool and method that I could find to impart information to my students. Pastors, counselors, and therapists not only present information to those who are battling fear and traumatic memories, but they also guide survivors through a minefield of deep emotional scars. This battle takes place in the survivors' minds and emotions.

Our emotions are controlled by our brains, and our brains are controlled by experiences, thoughts, and chemicals. We learn, and we can relearn. In essence, therapy is a classroom designed to aid in reconfiguring our thought processes to decrease stress levels and promote healing.

Interactive art is designed to be a graphic tool that can be used in the counselor's or individual's therapy session to help change a harmful mindset. If visual, auditory, reading/writing, and kinesthetic are the four methods used to aid in understanding and changing thought processes, each of these styles can be addressed by using a single interactive art print.

Who might benefit from using interactive art (IA) prints during individual, family, or group sessions?

- Counselors may find IA prints a powerful tool when treating victims of trauma, rape, robbery, and abuse of any type, including sexual, psychological, emotional, and physical abuse.
- Other clients, such as survivors of sex trafficking or prostitution, might release their thoughts, feelings, and emotional pain more readily when the therapist approaches them using an IA print.
- These prints can be used to counsel those dealing with racist wounds, family abuse, neglect and violence, death, divorce, issues of abandonment, PTSD, or depression, or any event that caused mental and emotional harm, distress, violence, or violation.
- Clients who are recovering from a single trauma event, chronic events, or multiple or complex events may benefit from using an interactive art print.
- Interactive art prints can be used by any age group, from childhood through adulthood.

Suggestions

The interactive art prints were created to be written on. The art is secondary to the information that it is holding. I have found that the best instrument to use for writing on the interactive art prints is a fine-point, black Sharpie permanent marker.

The author of this book, "Using Interactive Art as a Therapeutic Tool," gives permission for therapists to photocopy the interactive art prints from this book, giving an unlimited number of counseling session possibilities. All rights pertaining to the graphics and written text remain the property of the author, as stated on the copyright page of this book.

CHAPTER 3

Rooms in My Heart—Sadie's Story

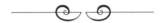

For many years, the original *Rooms in My Heart* (*RIMH*) design was just a rough sketch in a folder in my art room. But as with all tools, eventually you need to get them out and use them again. This was the case with my drawing and thoughts regarding the *RIMH* design.

One summer, I spent some time with a young father, his ten-year-old daughter, and the father's fiancée. The following are not their real names, but let's call them Drew, Sadie, and Kim, respectively. Sadie's birth mother and Drew were not together, but the mother was still alive and involved in Sadie's life. With her dad now engaged, I could see Sadie struggling to figure out how to respond to the new addition to her father's and her family. Sadie acted cold and aloof toward Kim, withholding friendship and any possibility of a relationship.

I remembered the *Rooms in My Heart* sketch I had made many years earlier to explain how I could love both of my husbands, differently yet equally. I knew I needed to put it into a visual that Sadie would understand, so I painted the original watercolor *RIMH*. Then I found a quiet moment to sit down with Sadie to talk about what she was feeling and to share this story.

It was the same story I'd shared with my friend many years ago. I told Sadie that we create a "room" in our heart for each person we know in our lifetimes. Each room is unique and special and can be filled with as much love and memories as we choose. I explained that she had a special space in her heart for her mother, but she had a room in her heart for her future stepmother. The two rooms were separate. She was not robbing love from one person when she gave love to another. We all need to give unlimited kindness and love and to make as many memories as time allows when we are with the person at that moment.

Sadie needed to see she was not betraying or stealing love from her mother by enjoying her time spent with her stepmother, and vice versa. She needed to understand that she would never run out of love to give. Her time spent with each occupant of a room created memories with that particular person, to be kept in their own places in her heart.

Again, the *RIMH* painting helped this young lady to recognize how and why she was feeling as she did, how to change that negativity, and how to move forward in a more positive attitude.

At the end of our chat, Sadie wore a wide grin as she said, "That's awesome! I get it! I really do!"

I could see the relief and change in her whole countenance. The idea that she had to choose whom to love was a burden that had weighed heavily on her. That burden was lifted when she realized she had plenty of love to share. She could see how that was possible because of the *RIMH* painting.

Again, *RIMH* can be used for so many more emotional struggles and wounds.

Uses: For melded families; children dealing with change in family dynamics; children and adults dealing with death or loss of family member or friend.

Karen E. Erdman, RN, BSN, MEd

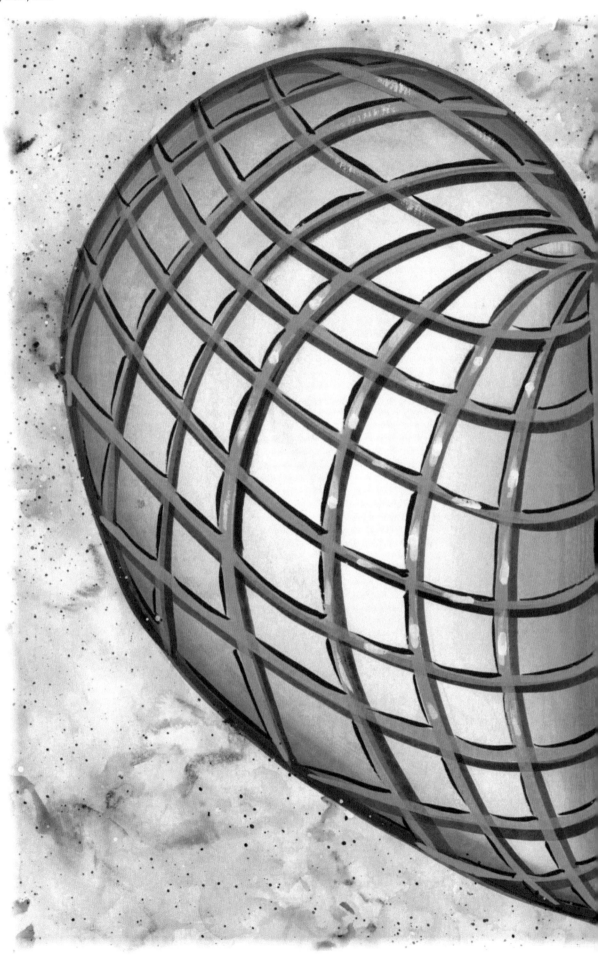

Interactive
Art Graphics
Number 1
*Rooms in
My Heart*

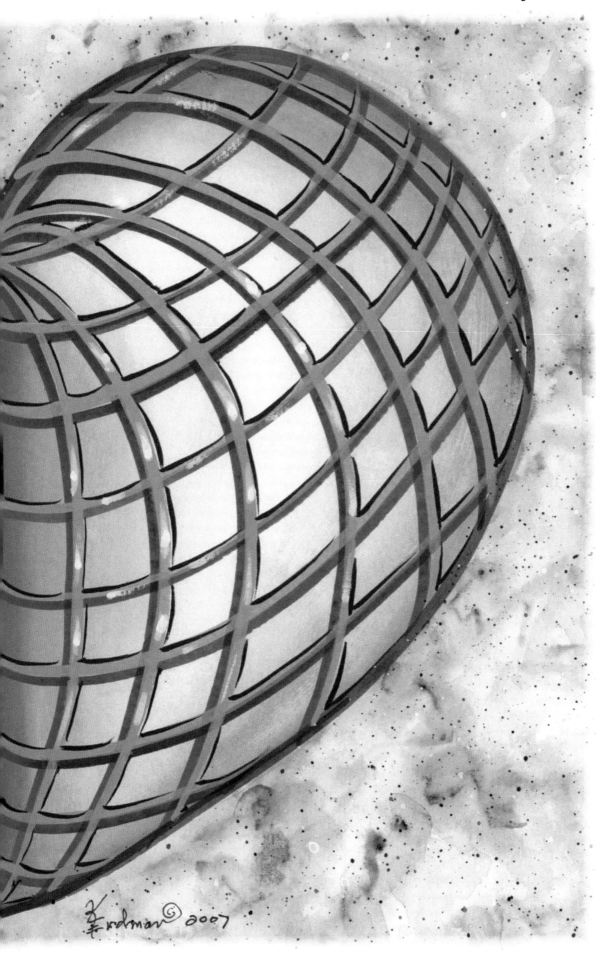

9

CHAPTER 4

Suggested Ways to Use Rooms in My Heart Print

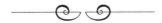

There are many ways to use the *Rooms in My Heart* print as a therapeutic aid in the healing process when dealing with loss or deep offense of almost any origin. The *RIMH* print is adaptable to the needs of the client.

For instance, if a client is dealing with the loss of a loved one, the therapist can invite the client to write the names of people that the client cares about, both living and dead, in the spaces of the heart. As the client writes the names on the print, the therapist can encourage the client to share specific memories of happy times spent with each room's occupant. When discussing a loved one who has passed away, the therapist can invite the client to remember and enjoy the feeling of being loved during those good memories of the loved one.

Even though they are separated by death, clients still are able to visit that special person with their hearts and minds, remembering good times, and knowing that the memories and love will remain with them. We cannot prevent people from dying, but we can continue to hold on to them in our hearts.

Another use for the interactive art (IA) print is to ask clients who experienced a tragic event or trauma, such as abuse, to fill in the rooms of the heart with the names of people they love and trust. They may choose to write positive events that had an affirmative impact on their lives. Maybe a teacher in third grade was the most influential person throughout their entire childhoods. Clients can list each specific time that they remember the teacher offering words of encouragement. They can choose to only list people's names or include all people, places, and/or events that affected them in a meaningful way.

The client and therapist may choose to limit the information written on the *RIMH* print to only include positive memories, or—this is the difficult part—the client can begin to fill in spaces that indicate a person, several people, one event, or multiple events that deeply scarred the client. The counselor, pastor, therapist, or social worker will guide the client to avoid retraumatization. The goal is not to relive the event but to recognize the feelings and thoughts the event caused. What is the present crisis to be addressed? The goal of using the IA prints is trauma resolution.

Counselors, clients, or individual persons, who are seeking healing by using the IA prints, can choose which method is best to *mark their hearts* in those areas that were or are painful from their past or present.

This will identify the areas where they hold the traumatic event(s). It's the wounded area in their hearts, so to speak.

Another suggestion would be to keep one room empty, signifying the person or event that caused the trauma. Clients may need to keep several rooms open because they have multiple hurts, people, and events that they need to address.

In identifying these areas of the heart that signify trauma, other options are to shade those areas in a different color to make it prominent or to write the name or initials of the offender (or the name of the place where the event happened), framed with colored edging. Maybe clients have experienced a traumatic occurrence such as a tornado, flood, earthquake, or fire. It is possible that certain colors indicate particular incidents to them. They can choose that specific color to signify the event on the print.

As the therapy sessions progress over time and when the client is ready, slowly, letter by letter, ask him or her to write a word such as *healed*, or *whole*, or *forgiven* in that space. Clients will see that the wounded part does not disappear. It remains a part of who they are, but hopefully, they will feel healing in those areas and see that the rest of their lives outshine the wounded areas. The goal is for the remaining positive areas of the heart to be more prominent and to overpower the once-all-consuming injured area(s) of their hearts.

Using an IA print to tangibly hold negative feelings, anger, thoughts, and fears, it can be placed at a position that is lower than or at a distance from the client, signifying to the brain that those negative thoughts are no longer a threat. With the help of the therapist, the client's brain hopefully will begin to recognize those negative feelings as nonthreatening.

Some people have suggested that these hurtful areas should be erased or whited out, which is something the client may choose to do. But in real life, with real feelings, that is not always possible. We cannot forget major tragedies and painful experiences. We can only fight to move through them and toward healing. Clients can strive to overcome the control that the wound and pain has had on their emotions, minds, and lives, but it still remains an element, a part of who they are. It is more likely that when clients see the area that has been branded *healed*, they will recognize that they can choose to be free from the control and oppression that the trauma has on their lives. It is a reminder of how far they have come and who they really are.

Examples of Other Causes of Emotional Damage Where IA Prints Can Be Used as a Healing Device: melded families; children dealing with change in family dynamics (divorce, parent deserted the family, parent sent to prison); children and adults dealing with death or loss of family members or friend; children and adults dealing with loss of any kind (feelings from loss of control, loss of property, loss of innocence, loss of physical well-being and safety); phobia and fear; career or family offenses

CHAPTER 5

Rooms in My Heart—Christian Perspective and Forgiveness

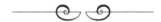

Not every therapist or client will use the interactive art prints based on a Christian foundation, but Christian therapists have used the prints numerous times. I will share the suggested manner that the *RIMH* print has been used in the past, based on a Christian platform.

First, at the beginning of most therapy sessions, it is beneficial to lead clients into a time to quiet their minds, relax, be still, and allow and promote a mental calmness. Invite the Holy Spirit's presence. When the client and the therapist both feel ready, move forward.

Second, ask the Holy Spirit to bring to the client's mind a remembrance of events and/or people who were and are a blessing—people who made the client feel stronger and secure; those who gave comfort and encouraged the client; people who made a positive impact in the client's life. Take the time to allow the client to reexperience those positive people and events. Direct the client to write those people's names in the spaces on the *RIMH* print as they come to mind. He or she can choose to write initials, names, places, or events. Do not hurry through this phase.

Repeat this search again and again, filling in the spaces, as well as around the heart, if needed. Take as much time as the client needs to fully appreciate each moment that adds a positive feeling of acceptance, friendship, protection, victory, accomplishments, warmth, encouragement, and love from his or her past.

Now comes the difficult part. Ask the client to mark the room or rooms that signify the traumatic event, or person who caused the client pain, or the place where the trauma occurred. As with so many trauma victims, clients relive feelings that the event caused, over and over. That is precisely why they seek help from professionals. Possibly, they have done the opposite and totally blocked out the memory. Encourage clients to close their eyes and ask God to help them truly admit to the fears and emotions they are experiencing. He may reveal the event to them and allow them to envision the event as it took place.

Only the therapist can decide what is best for each client. Retraumatization is a concern for many clients, and in that case, the therapist should ask clients only to identify what they feel. If they are in the event, tell them to invite the presence of Christ into that room. Ask them to visualize Jesus in the trauma with them. He was there all the time. He knows what they were and are feeling. Invite clients to envision Christ holding them. Instruct them to ask Jesus to help them heal and release that memory, that event, that pain into His hands.

Ask clients to write the letters J-e-s-u-s into the wounded space, writing one letter at a time, only as they feel a release from the past. It might take one, two, or three sessions, or it might take many, many sessions to begin to heal. Every person and every event they experience is unique. Each is deserving of one-to-one attention and focus from the clients themselves, from the therapist, and from God, who cares deeply about the wounds that are carried. When the process is complete, each person will have a graphic representation of how they released the memory into Christ's hands and healing.

Forgiveness—It is a Christian command and a crucial part of total healing.

> Forgive us our debts, as we have also forgiven our debtors. (Matthew 6:12 NIV)

Taking clients through sessions where they overcome painful past events eventually leads toward the prospect of forgiving those who were the perpetrators of the hurt. This might be the opportunity to complete the *RIMH* by whiting out or blocking out the wounded room as the client truly releases the anger.

I fell in love with the kids' definition from *Merriam-Webster Dictionary* for forgiveness: "The act of ending anger." Other words used in the adult definition are actions: "actively choosing release, to set free, ending, moving on."

On the Mayo Clinic's website, in the Healthy Lifestyle: Adult Health section, an article titled "Forgiveness: Letting go of grudges and bitterness" states the following:

> Letting go of grudges and bitterness can make way for improved health and peace of mind. Forgiveness can lead to healthier relationships, less stress, anxiety and hostility, lower blood pressure, and strengthen the immune system. (Mayo Clinic Staff 2020)

To choose to forgive is to:

- Make space for healing, love, and peace in the heart and mind of the client.
- Unlock the door to the room where hurt and bitterness have been held captive.
- Help overcome fear and anxiety.
- An anxious heart weighs a man down ... (Proverbs 12:25 NIV)
- Make room for more life as it was intended—joy, peace, and a closer relationship with God, family, and friends.

Without a doubt, it becomes work to push toward *not* crowding our lives and time with consuming thoughts of bitterness, fear, and anger that take the place of fulfillment and our true destiny in Christ in this world—the reason we are here on this planet. Unforgiveness is a self-destructive tool of Satan. Forgiveness is where the final stages of healing are found.

CHAPTER 6

Rooms in My Heart—Partners and Family

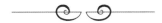

Partners

This chapter provides suggestions to counselors who provide couples therapy for partners in life or married couples. Any couple involved in a serious relationship who need help to repair wounds and hurts caused by themselves or others might benefit from the use of the *RIMH* print during counseling.

The Bible says, "And the two will become one flesh. So they are no longer two, but one" (Mark 10:8 NIV). Even science backs that statement with confirmation that when two people bond together, the chemical reaction is like a glue attachment in the brain.

In her article "The Science of Love and Attachment: How understanding your brain chemicals can help you build lasting love," Melanie Greenberg, PhD, states,

> Each stage in this cycle (lust, attraction, attachment) can actually be explained by your brain chemistry—the neurotransmitters that get you revved up and the hormones that carry the feelings throughout your body. According to anthropology professor Helen Fisher, there are three stages of falling in love. In each stage, a different set of brain chemicals run the show. (3-30-2016)

When partners have difficulties and consider separation or divorce, there are physical and chemical reactions that cause emotional stress, pain, and intense feelings, especially if it is coupled with betrayal and rejection.

During a therapy session with partners or couples, the *RIMH* is one heart, but it can be shared by two people. "The two shall be come one" (Mark 10:8 NIV). During a therapy session, each partner can choose a side of the IA heart and write in the spaces all the good things he or she remembers about their relationship, and then use another color to write in the negative events or hurts that have caused pain to him or her. As the hurtful areas on the heart are addressed, the client who has written those words on the IA heart can decide to write over that area with words such as *forgiven, new, faith,* or *renewed;* if the client chooses, it can be erased.

If a couple decides to part ways, it is like the heart is torn in two. Just like the paper of the *RIMH* print, it cannot be easily repaired. Tape can pull the sides together, but it will never be like it was before the split. The tearing away from each other, like the paper print, will never be as it was before it was marred. The mended area is a sign to the couple that their relationship was worth fighting for and that they did indeed work through difficult emotions.

Through the counselor, the couple hopefully will be able to take responsibility for their own parts in the marriage problems, embrace forgiveness, make a plan together for healing their relationship, and move on with a whole heart again, as partners in life.

Family

During a family therapy session, members of the family can write down all their names in the spaces of the *RIMH* print. They can include everyone in the family, both dead and alive, who have made an impact on and memories with them. The family can discuss their feelings for everyone whose name is written in the heart and the love they share for one another. They also can talk about when to let someone find his or her own path in life, but that does not mean that person is not part of the family or that the love that the family has for him or her ever stops.

Sometimes, certain family members were not a blessing but more like an evil curse. Each member of the family may have different memories of that specific family member. Honesty, acceptance, and support of each person's experience is important, as that allows each person to share his or her true feelings with the family. In this case, each member of the family may choose a specific color to signify the person who has caused harm to other family members. The therapist can then work through sessions, targeting feelings of betrayal, abandonment, abuse, and so on.

If the therapy is an intervention, such as a drug intervention, this visual may help the client see that he or she is part of the whole family. Family members and supporters would each write their names in a block of the *RIMH*. They also could write in the names of those who were unable to be present but who are equally involved and concerned for the client.

As the client views the *RIMH* print, the therapist reminds the client that the human heart does not function properly, if at all, when any part of the heart is missing, damaged, malfunctioning, or hurting. A heart attack is painful for everyone, so clients aren't just damaging themselves; they are hurting the whole family, the whole heart.

Group

There may be times when a group therapy is warranted, such as during a natural catastrophe or group trauma such as a school shooting. Group survivors of tornados, mudslides, floods, violent events, physical assaults, and racial violence may benefit from mutual survivor support during therapy. Client conversations in group therapy would focus on their deepest fears and feelings, which can be written on the *RIMH* print. There is strength in seeing that they all feel the same emotions. They all share the same survivor camaraderie. The counselor can direct the discussion to fight survivor's guilt by using the *RIMH* print.

CHAPTER 7

Other Prints as Therapeutic Tools

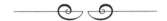

The Wisdom Tree—Positive Words of Affirmation

Blessed are those who find wisdom ... she is a tree of life to those
who embrace her; happy are those who hold her tightly.
—Proverbs 3:13–18 (NIV)

The Wisdom Tree print can be used several different ways. One suggestion would be to give the print to clients to keep in their homes. Instruct clients to write positive and encouraging words, sayings, poems, song lyrics, scriptures, or anything else that is uplifting to them on the print. These words can help clients who battle depression to focus on feeling brighter and more positive. They can hang the print in an area where they will see it often. If there was a special person in their lives who had a favorite saying or quote, clients can write that on the print. These should be constructive words that build up their thinking and emotions. The combination of a special statement plus the feeling of being cared for could be enough to get clients through another day while at home.

Alternately, while the print may be used as described above, it can also be kept in the therapist's office instead of the client's home. Then, at each session, clients would be asked to add to *The Wisdom Tree* those words that have meaning and insight into their healing processes.

Those who are dealing with feelings of low self-esteem can write uplifting words or declarations of who they really are, not what they have experienced in the past. They can declare that they are now survivors and not victims. Therapists can invite clients to say those words that are written on *The Wisdom Tree* out loud as a confirmation of who they really are. Share this statement: "If you *leaf* those thoughts to take *root*, those thoughts will *branch* out to become *oak tree*–sized attitudes!" (Corny, I know.)

One last suggestion for using *The Wisdom Tree* is for the client to write positive words in a themed manner; he or she would find and write down all appropriate scriptures that talk about, for example, battling fear. Other subjects that may be appropriate are love, strength, healing, protection, joy, peace, or self-control.

Tread On—A Visual List of Steps

This print encourages the client to move forward and walk on in life. It could be used as a tangible reminder of each new accomplishment the client attains. They should set goals by writing them in the steps on the print, then walk into the process of achieving them. Whether the person is struggling with obsessive-compulsive behavior or post-traumatic stress disorder, this print would be a reminder of each solid step forward that the client makes.

Tread On might be a visual log of planned or unplanned achievements attained if the client is dealing with fear or PTSD. The client could fill in each step with goals that combat a certain fear. For example, clients can make a list of goals, and write each goal on a step. As clients meet each goal, they can write the date it was achieved or cross off the goal with a large marker. As an example, the client who is a rape survivor would write goals that would help to fight those crippling thoughts and feelings. Some ideas to write on the steps as goals are to see a therapist, take self-defense classes, buy pepper spray, change security systems, or work on creating different routes to get to work. Again, this is a visual confirmation that they are moving forward in their lives, and they are gaining control over their lives again.

Fallen Leaves—Events to "Leaf" Behind

This print signifies the events that the client wants to purge from his or her memory. During the therapy session, each time the client brings up a hurt, fear, or struggle, he or she would write it in a leaf. The client would work through these issues with the counselor during the therapy sessions. At the last session, the client can burn the print, signifying the release from those struggles.

This print can be used in a group or milieu therapy, with possibly every client writing one goal to achieve before the next session. To encourage accountability, post the print where clients can be reminded of the goals they set.

Salvation—Place It on the Cross

Sometimes counselors help clients who are perpetrators, rather than victims or survivors. For the Christian, the death and Resurrection of Jesus Christ says it all and means everything. It is where God's fullness of grace and humankind's redemption exist. These clients may also be victims of their own personal hurts or incidents from their pasts that caused them to be filled with rage and resentment. If clients seek healing and forgiveness, their writing those events and emotions on the *Salvation* cross may begin the healing that the perpetrators need to understand in order to stop hurting other people. Clients might never have experienced the freedom of letting go of their own pain and guilt.

Party Balloons—A Cause for Celebration! (Two print choices: a *nine*- or *fifteen*-balloon print)

These prints may be just the visual to which a young or young-at-heart client can relate. There are two clouds above the balloons. In those clouds, clients might choose to write their names in one cloud, and You Are Loved in the other—or possibly something like, You Are an Achiever or My Talents. Encourage users to celebrate who God made them to be.

In the balloons, the therapist can direct clients to write past achievements, pleasant memories, friends, teachers, talents, or people and happy events that lifted their spirits and made them feel special. The therapist might suggest using each balloon to represent a specific time in the client's life.

Like chapters in a book, each balloon might indicate a certain timeline. Encourage clients to remember that a story might start off tragic, but they are in charge of how their stories proceed and end. They have the authority to determine the nature of their life stories. They can choose to head toward an ending that is victorious and filled with restoration, joy, and blessings. They can hang on to the positive helium-filled balloons and let go of the deflated balloons that hold them down.

They also can write on the ribbons. They might write long-term goals on the balloons and short-term goals on the ribbons; they might write events on the balloons and people's names along the ribbons.

Label Me Bright—Looking Forward in Life; Change Your Label

One of my favorite seafood meals is centered on fresh flounder broiled in butter. If you've never eaten fresh flounder fillet, you are missing a wonderful treat. But I digress. An adult flounder has two eyes, just like many of God's creatures, but an adult flounder is a bottom-dweller that has two eyes on one side of its body, specifically the top side. It can see its prey coming as it lies at the bottom of the ocean. The flounder has a built-in protection system because of the positioning of its eyes.

Human eyes, on the other hand, are on the front of our heads, which enables us to walk forward and see where we are going. We don't do very well if we walk backward because we can't see what is behind us. If we lived our lives walking backward, we would constantly stumble and fall.

My suggestion for using *Label Me Bright* is to plan forward and upward thinking. Encourage clients to write where they want to go in life—possible achievements they want to move forward and upward toward.

Clients also can use this print to write each achievement they accomplish each day or possibly each week. The success could be:

- Made lunch for myself.
- Completed most [or all] of my homework.
- Got through one day without a single fight.
- Made it through three days straight without having any arguments with my parents.

Now, that's looking good with both eyes focused forward in a positive manner!

Either the *Party Balloons* or *Label Me Bright* print could be used to aid a youth in creating a register—keeping a Responsibility Chart to list ongoing actions that signify the ability to take on responsibility. The client would be asked to write the expected act in one area (balloon or label), then keep a tally, with an X signifying each time he or she completes that activity. The timeline would be set by the therapist and client, whether one week or one month, for projected logging of each activity. For example,

Week One
Made my bed XXXXX
Cleaned my room X
Took trash out XX
Completed homework XXXXXX

Sticks and stones will break bones, and words really do hurt. For children or adolescents, it is hurtful when other people label them in ways that destroy their self-esteem. Parents or friends can be responsible for unwittingly attaching the wrong label to a child or youth. Invite children or teens to relabel themselves. Ask them to discuss and list how they can take control of their labels and change them.

Camouflage—Hidden Hindrances

What are the destructive, harmful habits, addictions, or traits that clients are struggling to admit to themselves or others, which causes them to falter in life? Using the *Camouflage* print to identify and discuss those oppressions with a counselor may be the tool they need to attain relief from the burden of those life choices. How does one erase the damage to relationships, guilt, and shame that frequently accompanies harmful practices? Face them. Address them. Acknowledge that they are there. Then, with the guidance of a therapist, clients can work toward freeing themselves from those crippling bondages. Upon completion of the therapy sessions, clients may choose to destroy the print by burning it or shredding it. This can signify to clients that they are released from those harmful habits.

Suggestions for using the *Camouflage* print are as follows:

1. When the client discloses to the therapist specific, undesirable behaviors, the therapist can ask the client to write them on the print. It could be something like a battle with pornography, drug abuse, abusive behaviors, anger, or alcohol abuse.
2. Throughout the following sessions the client can write around the behavior any triggers, secret practices, or excuses used that would support the continuation of the controlling conduct.
3. Around those triggers and practices, the client or therapist can discuss and write down possible solutions and ways to avoid and combat those triggers that would lead the client back into the center of the harmful behaviors. Identify the battle, then formulate the plan to win.

Karen E. Erdman, RN, BSN, MEd

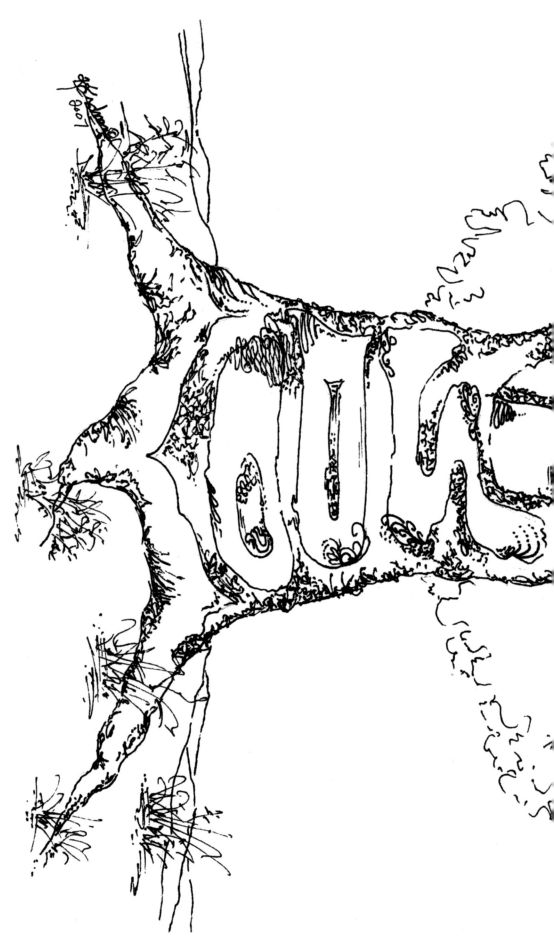

Interactive
Art Graphics
Number 2
*The Wisdom
Tree*

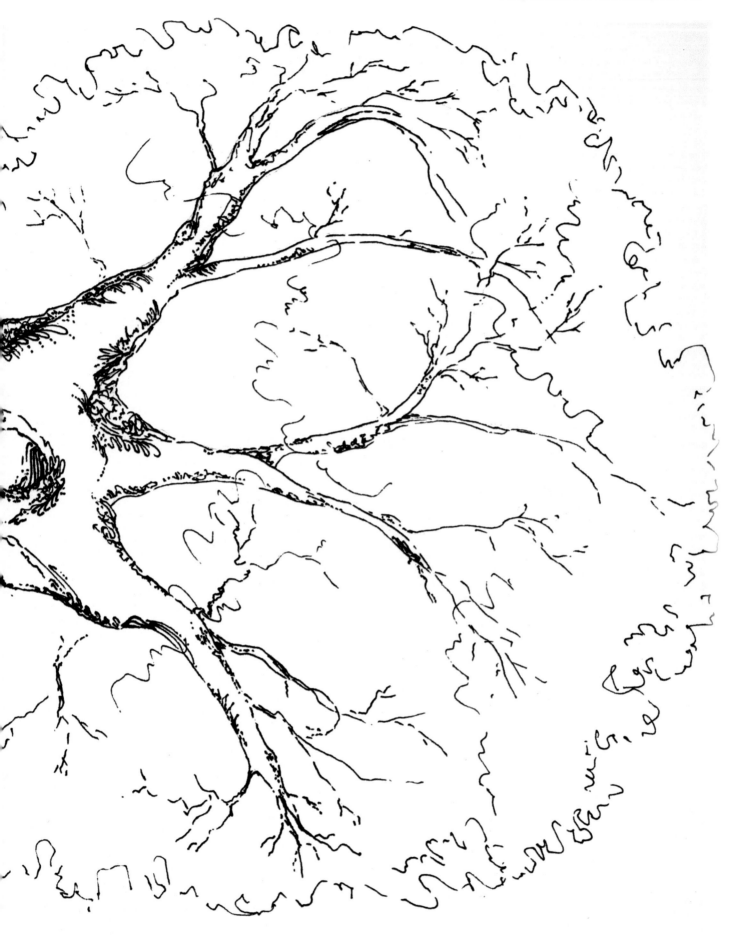

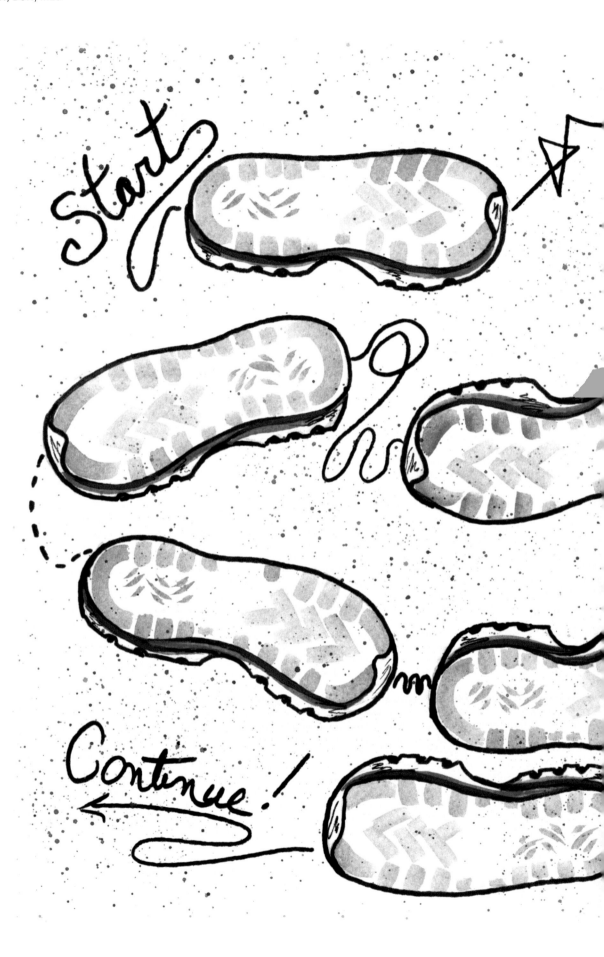

Interactive
Art Graphics
Number 3
Tread On

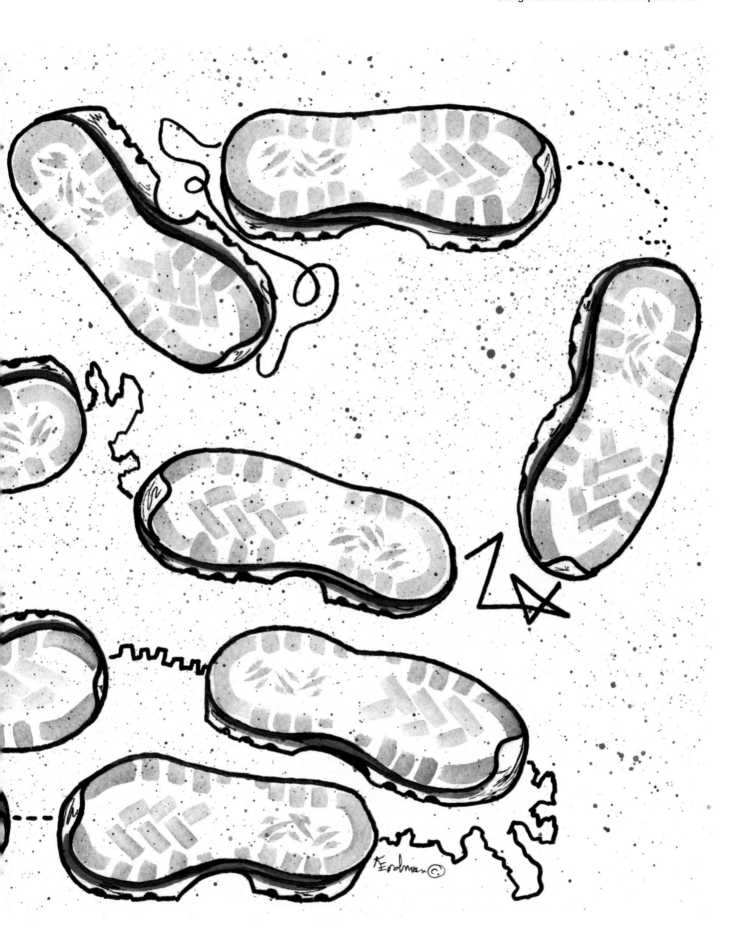

Interactive
Art Graphics
Number 4
Fallen Leaves

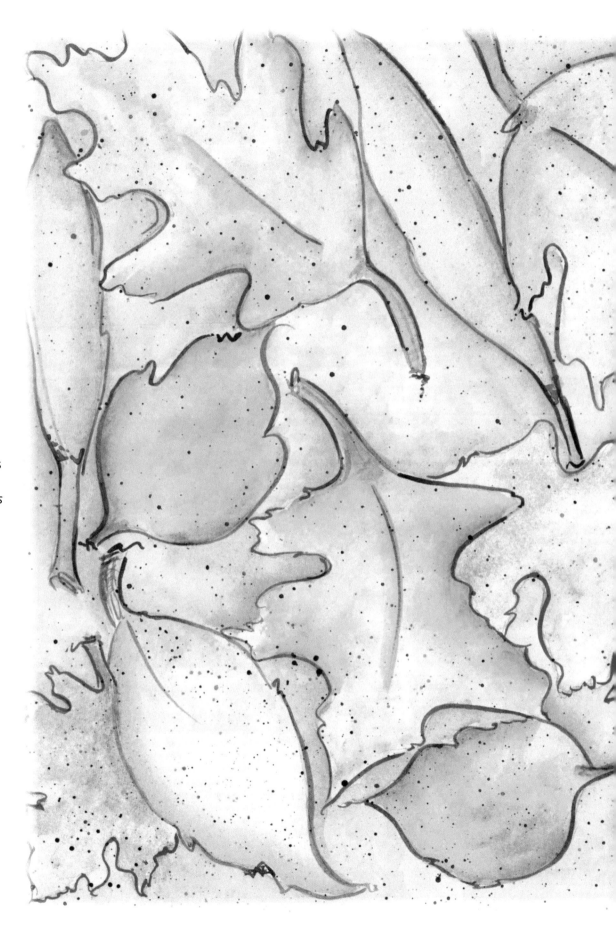

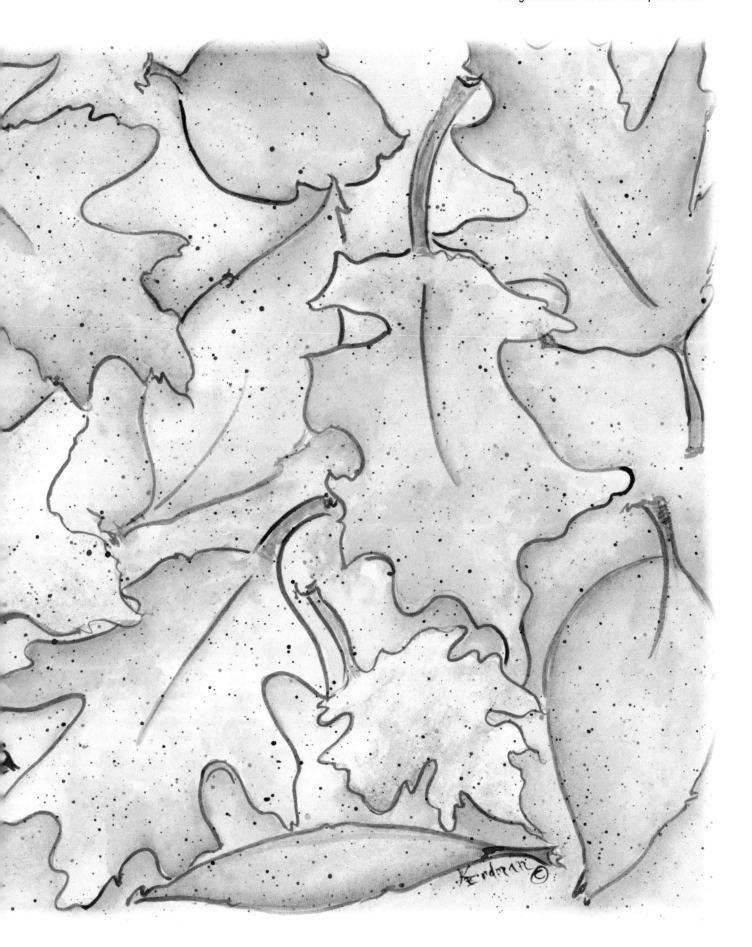

Karen E. Erdman, RN, BSN, MEd

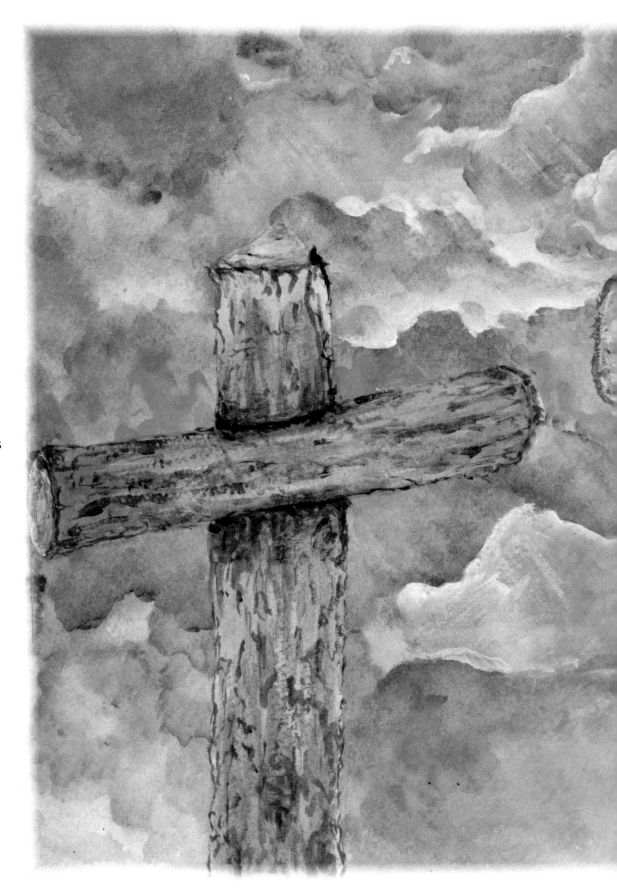

Interactive
Art Graphics
Number 5
Salvation

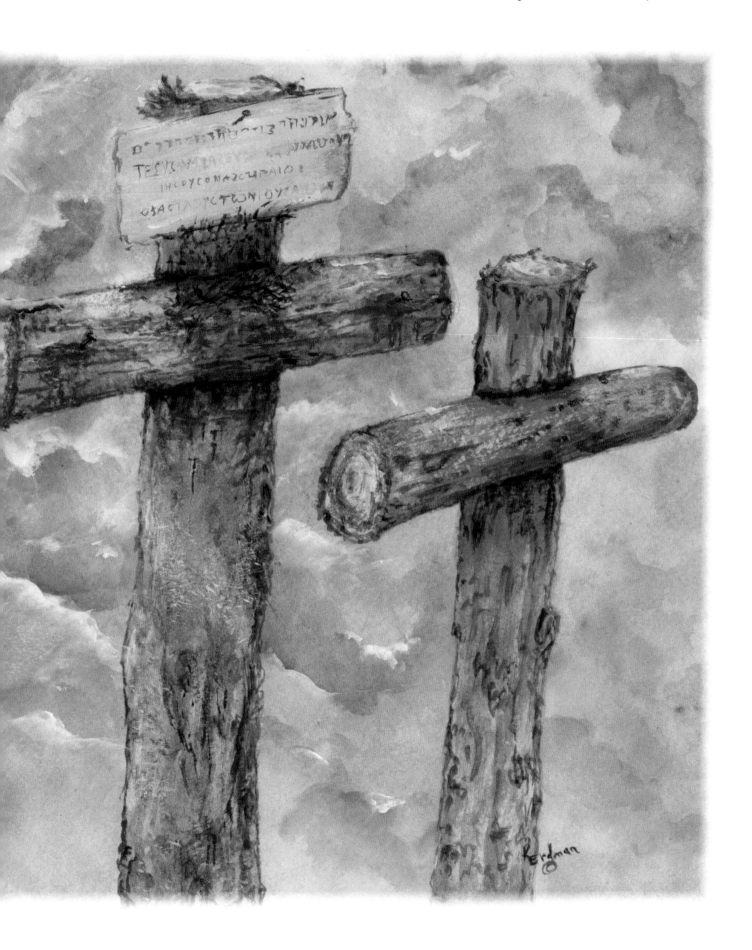

Interactive
Art Graphics
Number 6
*Party
Balloons* (15)

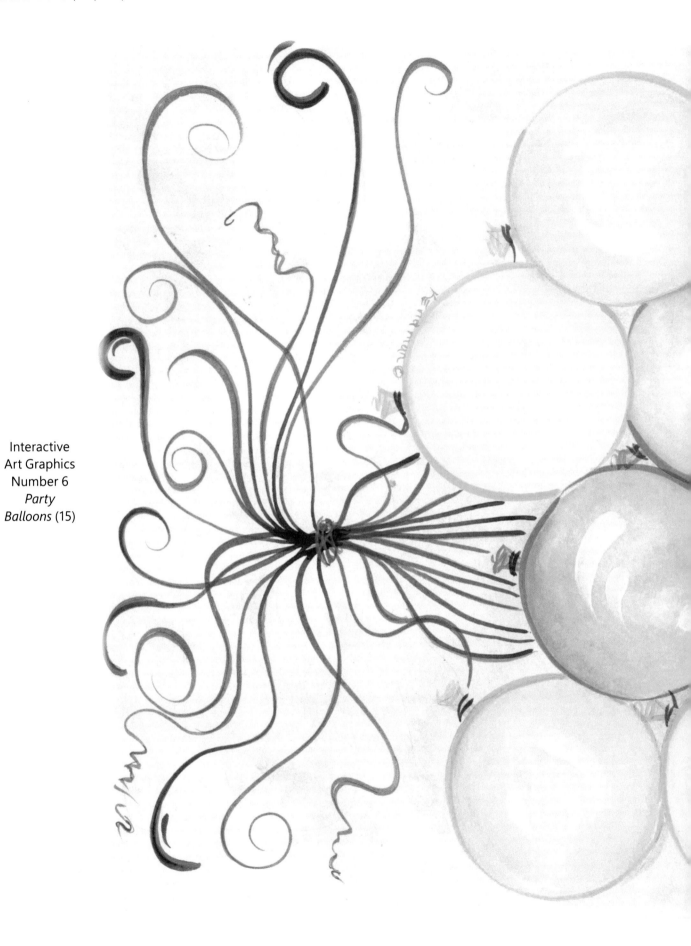

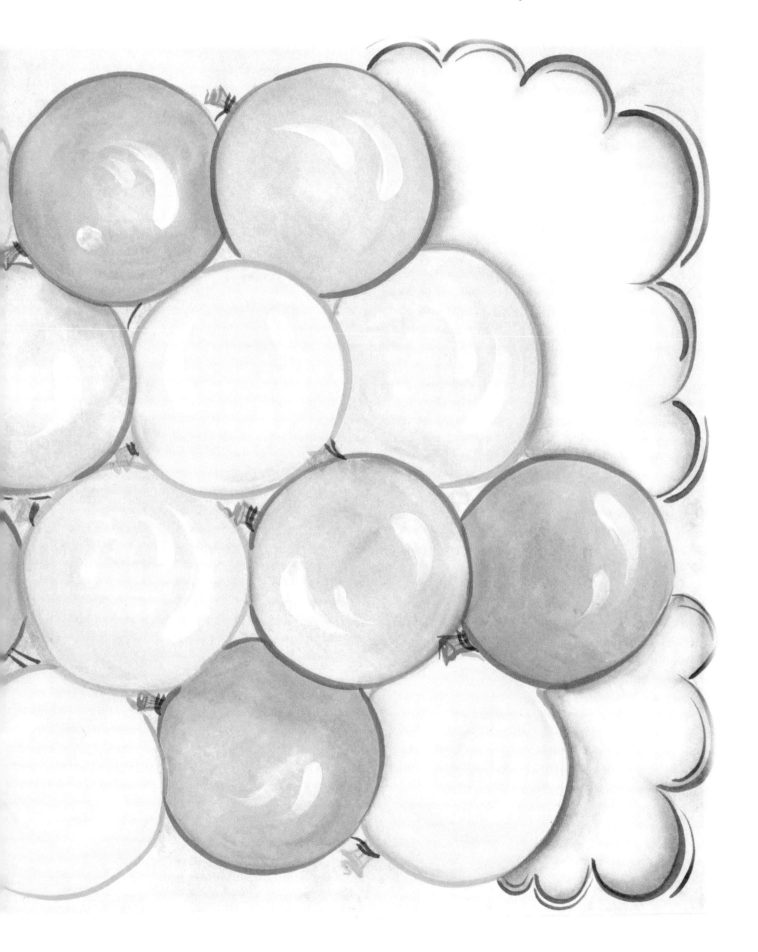

Interactive
Art Graphics
Number 7
*Party
Balloons* (9)

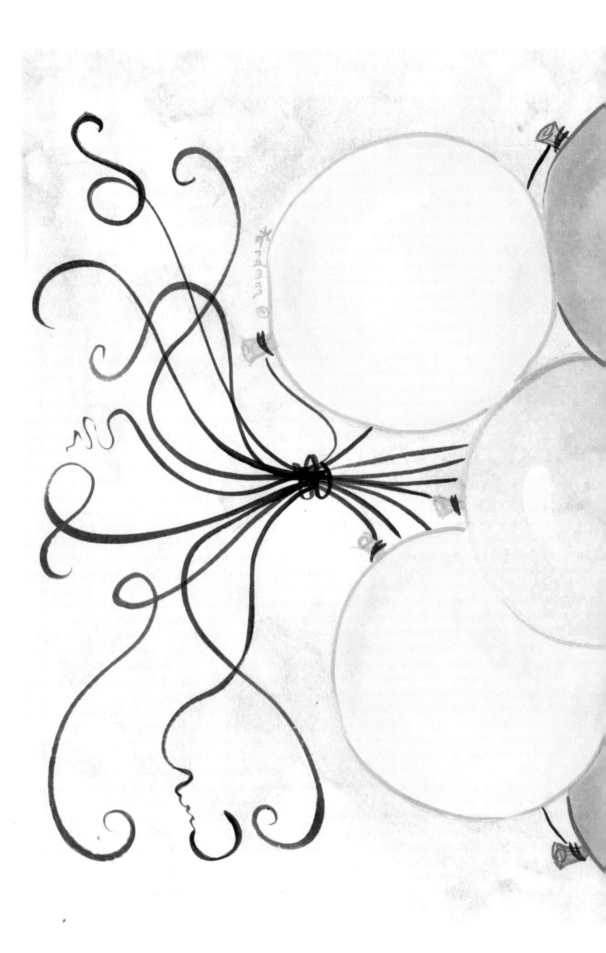

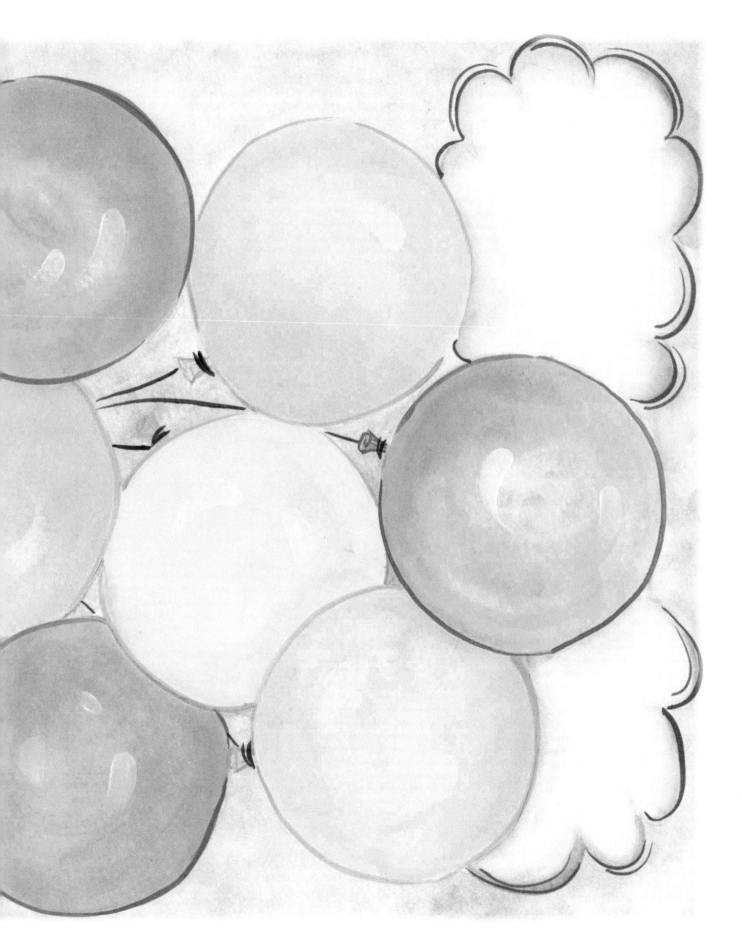

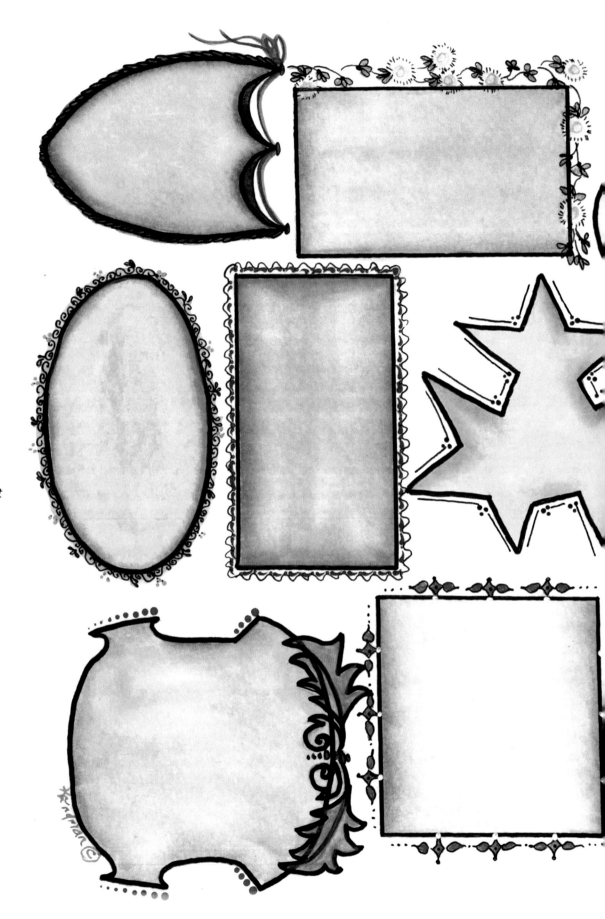

Interactive
Art Graphics
Number 8
Label Me Bright

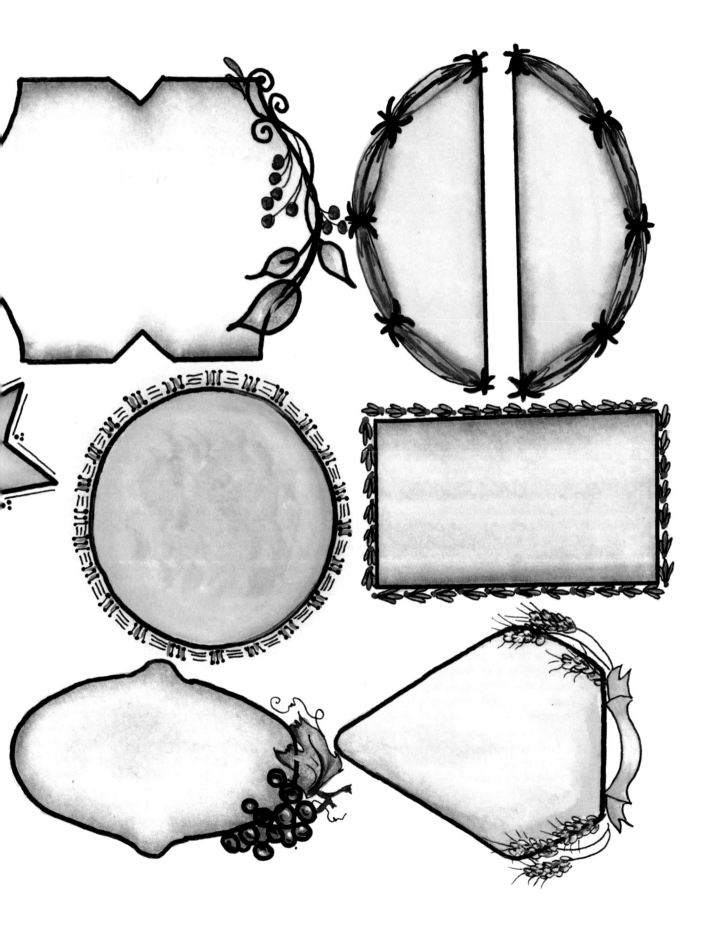

Karen E. Erdman, RN, BSN, MEd

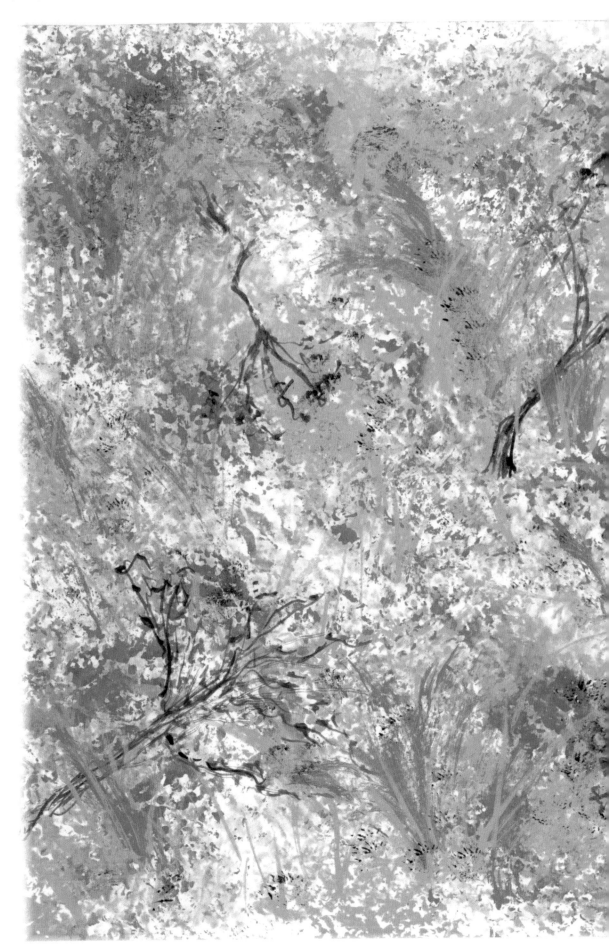

Interactive
Art Graphics
Number 9
Camouflage

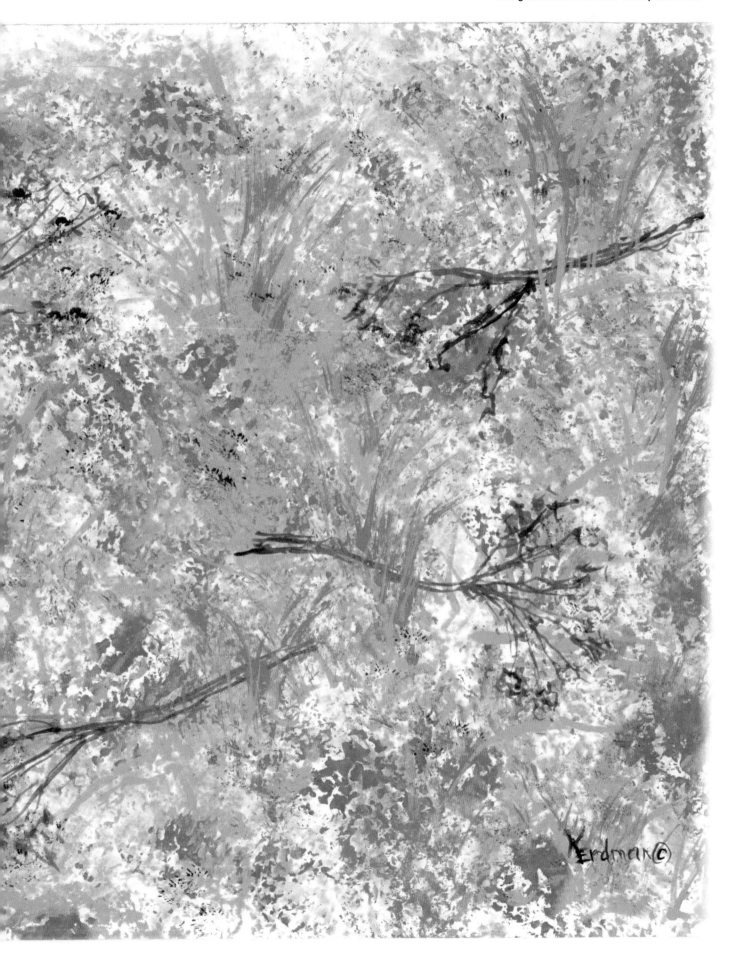

CHAPTER 8

Testimony

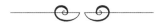

A therapist can use the interactive art prints in so many ways during therapeutic sessions or home assignments. Each client and his or her experiences are unique. Like any medical condition, the treatment needs to be personalized. Only the therapist will know how to use the prints to achieve optimum results with each client. The therapist will know each client's needs, willingness, history, and responsiveness to the therapy tool.

The following is a testimony from a friend who used the *RIMH* print to address heart wounds from her past. She altered and adapted the method of using the *RIMH* print to suit her own needs.

She wrote the following:

> Karen and I were friends when she first introduced me to her interactive art. I loved the concept and immediately purchased her *Wisdom Tree* to hang on the wall of my home and invite guests to write and share wisdom as they visited. I also bought *Fallen Leaves* for my son and his wife to record their hikes and adventures because they are very outdoorsy. Finally, I purchased *The Traveler* for my daughter who is the world trekker of the family.
>
> Years later, I found myself in a place where I knew that I needed some spiritual, emotional, and psychological healing. Decades of wounds seemed to have accumulated, creating a burden and a roadblock in my life. While I thought I had forgiven and put these issues to rest, somehow these things were still hindering me, still rearing their ugly heads, still consuming my thoughts. After spending time in prayer, I realized that I needed to commit to a deeper work of healing, and the Lord led me to Karen's *Rooms in My Heart*. Jesus has used this beautiful tool to take me on an authentic cleansing and healing journey.
>
> Karen's gift of artistry and her compassionate heart, coupled with the love, wisdom, and healing power of the Holy Spirit, have produced a therapeutic tool that enables breakthrough and transformation. *Rooms in My Heart* has been life changing. It has lifted burdens and brought forgiveness and freedom to my life.
>
> There may be many ways you could use this tool, so in addition to reading the instructions in this book, I encourage you to pray and allow the Holy Spirit to guide you. In my case, I wrote in each box (or room) of the heart those things that caused me spiritual, emotional, or psychological pain—things like a person's name, a particular topic or issue, or a memory. This took several days. When I felt I had everything down on paper that was presently troubling me, I focused on one issue at a time, really praying through it

and seeking the Lord for healing. I allowed Him to direct me to scripture. I allowed Him to speak, and I journaled quite a bit as He spoke to me throughout my healing journey.

As I began to experience a little healing, I wrote a J (for Jesus) with a pink highlighter over top of that issue. After a bit more healing came, I wrote E, until I eventually had written *JESUS*. Then, as a bit more healing came, I underlined the word *JESUS* and drew a line over top (still with the pink highlighter). Finally, only as I got to a place where I felt that particular issue lift off me, where I was completely released from it and experienced peace, I colored that block entirely pink with the highlighter. The pink highlighter was symbolic to me as it reminded me of the pink color of a scar where a wound had recently healed. Some blocks took many hours, days, and even weeks of prayer and time with the Lord before I could color them completely pink. Others took only a few minutes.

Over time, I wrote more issues in vacant blocks. It seemed that when one issue was healed, another bubbled up. Sometimes, when focusing on a particular topic, related issues came to my mind. I didn't ignore any of them. If something bubbled up, I wrote it down so I could deal with it.

I also wrote positive words in some of the empty rooms—things that I wanted to walk in or be; things that I wanted to be a part of my core; godly things like joy, faith, peace, wisdom, hope, love, purity, humility, etc. I also wrote positive words or statements about areas where I was struggling. For example, I wrote, *I have something to offer*, and *valued*, *complete*, *bold*, *worthy*, and more. Again, I prayed into each of these things. As I began to feel the Lord's loving affirmations to me in these areas, once again, over time, I wrote *JESUS*, but this time I wrote in a blue highlighter. And when I truly believed that I had received these beautiful gifts from the Lord, I colored them fully in blue highlighter. For me, this symbolized the living water of the Lord Jesus.

Over time, I wrote, in the margins of the heart, beautiful affirmations from the Lord—areas where perhaps I'd wavered or doubted and needed to be reminded. I wrote things like, *I am secure in Jesus; I am adequate in Jesus; I am loved by Jesus; I am loveable because He created me; He chose me; He called me; I am important to Jesus; I am valued by Jesus*. I also wrote simple prayers in the margins, like, *Bind up my wounds. Apply healing balm, salve, ointment*. I declared scripture in the margins, such as, *By His stripes, I am healed*.

This heart print became a keepsake of precious time spent with my Lord. It is also proof of my healing. *Rooms in My Heart* has taken me on quite the emotional journey. I have cried many tears. It was painful to relive some things, but it was also freeing to get to the roots and deal with them completely. It didn't happen quickly, yet I absolutely wanted to invest the time that I needed to be free so that I could be all the Lord is calling me to be without hindrances from the past.

There is not one speck of space left on the print to write anything else; I have completely filled it. At times, I have even drawn separate hearts on different pieces of paper when a particular issue was rather deep, with many layers that I had to sort through.

To date, the heart still has some uncolored areas, some issues where the wounds are too fresh or too deep or complex for me to color them in fully yet. There are also other things written in blocks that I haven't completed yet, simply because they are future goals, such as books or blogs that I still want to write and other goals that I am still working toward, such as health goals.

While this print represents my journey of tears, it also showcases the beauty that comes from knowing that I have forgiven others, and I have been forgiven. I have healed, and I am now free. It's a beautiful tapestry of the Lord's love and a demonstration of hours of time spent together with my Savior, who loves me more than anyone on this planet.

If those pesky issues try to nag at me again, I simply will roll open this heart and gaze upon it, drinking in the memories. I will remember my journey and remind myself that I have dealt with this. I am healed, free, and whole. Joy is my companion.

At the very center of my heart, I have written these words: *Jesus Heals and Restores*. After all, that's the central point of it all.

Thank you, Karen, for being the hands and feet of Jesus and offering this wonderful, Holy Spirit–inspired healing tool.

And, dear reader, may God richly bless you in your healing journey.

CHAPTER 9

Message to the Reader

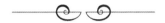

I dream almost every night. Sometimes my dreams are fairly long. Some dreams are skits, and some are snippets of who knows what. In some dreams I have no clue what I am thinking or seeing; they make no sense. Other dreams are a result of something I am feeling emotionally, and it shows up in a dream. Yet there are other dreams that I am quite certain are God's message to me. For those dreams, I simply allow God to reveal the meaning to me after I am awake. Sometimes I understand the meaning of the dream right away, and sometimes He shows me the significance of the dream later.

One dream I had was vivid while I was dreaming, and I still can see it in my mind. This was my dream:

A large group of people were standing to my left. In front of all of us was a gray stone wall, about four feet wide and two feet high. On top of this wall was a large window frame made of a light aluminum-type material. There was no glass in it, just the large square frame. The people were all carrying bundles wrapped in grayish material. Each person had a different sized bundle—some small, some large. They had the choice to carry the bundle around the wall or to throw their bundles through the open window. When the people tossed their bundles through the window, the bundles "riced" or dispersed into tiny fragments. Then they would walk around the wall without the parcel.

In my dream, I knew the people were never forced to throw their bundles through the window; I knew they had a choice. They were free to walk around the wall, carrying their bundles, and move on with their lives, although they would be weighed down by their bundles; or they could toss the bundle through the window, and it would be pulverized. No one made them choose either option. But I also knew that when they were bundle-free, there was a lightness to them, and they were so much happier. That is where the dream ended, and I woke up.

I interpreted the dream to mean that people have the choice to throw their burdens through to Jesus, and He will take them and dissolve them. I also felt that the dream was significant to the interactive prints and their uses.

A short time later, I was praying with one of my prayer partners. I asked her to pray for the interactive art therapy book. I also shared this dream with her.

She said, "It's about the graphic designs! They are meant for people to throw their painful traumas, past hurts, and present struggles to Jesus, using the interactive art as a 'windowna'."

This leads to my final thoughts for you, the reader.

My sincere hope is that God will use the written information and graphic designs from this therapeutic-tool workbook to stir your thought processes. My desire is that it will assist those who dedicate their lives to others by way of therapy and counseling. It is a gift to have this insight into mending hearts and lives. May God lead and bless you as you minister to others.

Also, if you are an individual who is looking for a method to release past injuries, my wish is that this book will lead you forward into rebuilding your life and letting go of past wounds. Blessings to you as you move toward restoration and healthful living!

CHAPTER 10

The Amen Chapter

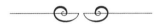

I titled this chapter "The Amen Chapter" because it is the end of the book, yet it might be a new beginning for you. I do not have eloquent words to share with you, just the truth that God gives from His Word.

If you do not have a real, live, working, daily, intimate relationship with Christ, this is a great day to start. A life walking with God is a life filled with adventures beyond your wildest dreams. And that life lasts for an eternity.

Who?

Who should invite Jesus into their lives?

For God so loved *the world* that he gave his only Son, that *whoever* believes in him should not perish but have eternal life. (John 3:16 KJV, italics added)

Why?

1. You will know that you are saved.
2. God loves you and wants a personal relationship with you.

Then you will call upon me and come and pray to me and I will hear you. You will seek me and find me; when you seek me with all your heart. (Jeremiah 29:12,13 KJV)

And you will know the truth, and the truth will make you free. (John 8:32 KJV)

When?

He is calling to you now!

I pray that the eyes of your heart may be enlightened in order that you may know the hope to which he has called you, the riches of his glorious inheritance in his holy people, and his incomparably great power for us who believe. (Ephesians 1:18–19 NIV)

You are a chosen race, a royal priesthood, a holy nation, a people for God's own possession, so that you may proclaim the excellencies of Him who has called you out of the darkness into His Marvelous light. (1 Peter 2:9 KJV)

How?

It is as simple as A-B-C.

Admit you are a sinner.

Since all have sinned and fall short of the glory of God … (Romans 3:23 KJV)

Believe Jesus is who He says He is.

Therefore, God has highly exalted Him and bestowed on Him the name which is above every name, that at the name of Jesus every knee should bow in heaven and on the earth, and under the earth, and every tongue confess that Jesus Christ is Lord, to the glory of God the Father. (Philippians 2:9–11 KJV)

Confess Jesus as your Savior. Invite Him into your life.

Because, if you confess with your lips that Jesus is Lord and believe in your heart that God raised Him from the dead, you will be saved. (Romans 10:9 KJV)

What?

What do you do now?

- Be all in. You do not have to worry about changing; let God work on you. *Be willing* to yield to His will.
- Find a good, solid, *Bible-believing church* to help guide and support your spiritual growth.
- *Tell someone*, such as a pastor or Christian friend, that you received salvation and that you are now a child of God.
- *Pray.* (That is simply talking with God.)
- Keep *listening* for His voice. He *is* there with you.
- Get a Bible that you can understand—perhaps the New International Version (NIV)—and *read.* Maybe start with Psalms and Proverbs and then the New Testament (Matthew, Mark, Luke, John, etc.).

Welcome to the Family of God!

The Lord bless you and keep you; The Lord make His face to shine upon you and be gracious to you; The Lord lift up His countenance upon you and give you peace.
(Numbers 6:24–26 KJV)

Suggested Reading

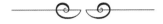

The first two books listed are page-turners. Anyone who reads either of these books will not be disappointed. Each has a message that will mesmerize the reader, and each has a healing message. The first book is fiction, and the second book is nonfiction.

I have read and highly recommend the following books:

Healing from Abortion

Deborah Arlene, *The Dream* (Meadville, PA: Christian Faith Publishing, Inc., 2019).

Abortion doesn't just destroy the life of the fetus. Abortion destroys the peace and lives of the child's parents. For those who are dealing with postabortion grief, read this novel. It leads the reader through the difficult topic of abortion in a most loving and caring manner. Therapists who counsel women postabortion (and men) can offer this book without fear of seeming to condemn or preach. It is filled with grace, support, hope, and healing. This book might well be the salve that breaks through to the underlying wound in the lives of those who suffer from postabortion trauma.

Healing from Abuse

Sarah Isaac-Samuel, *A Journey Back to Restoration* (Naples: Powerful You! Inc. USA Publishing, 2018).

Countless people in this world are hurting because of their past traumas. Author Sarah Isaac-Samuel shares her personal story—from hopelessness and helplessness to victory through God's healing power. In this present space in time, when so many damaged people are looking to make that same journey out of darkness, this book is filled with encouragement. It is a testimony of how one woman headed toward the light of hope, even when there seemed to be none. Without a doubt, it is an emotional, no-holds-barred testimonial that truly points to God's hand of deliverance and restoration.

Critically Needed and Unique Genre: Understanding, Ministering to, and Supporting Missionaries

Lois A. Dodds, PhD, and Laura Mae Gardner, DMin, *Global Servants, Cross-Cultural Humanitarian Heroes, Volume 1: Formation and Development of These Heroes* (Liverpool, PA: Heartstream Resources, Inc., 2010).

Note: This book's birth, construction, and content was written in part by two beloved colleagues of the authors, whose passing during the writing of this book was profoundly felt—Lawrence E. Dodds, MD, MPH (husband of Dr. Lois Dodds) and Mary Lazarides, MDiv.

This is a three-volume series.

None of the altruistic directives that Bible scriptures give us can be carried out by accident.

> They must be deliberately addressed by nations, organizations, and individuals—our cross-cultural humanitarian heroes. This book is concerned with the care of those global servants. We want to share the perspectives, principles, and strategies which will allow humanity's special servants to go beyond merely surviving the rigors and challenges to thriving. (Dodds and Gardner 2010, xi)

Dr. Lois Dodds is president and director of Heartstream Resources, Inc., a nonprofit agency that serves the needs of humanitarian workers around the globe. Her work has included personnel selection and training and psychological assessment of candidates for overseas work. With her husband, the late Lawrence Dodds, MD, she devoted decades to caring for these special global servants through counseling, residential treatment programs, retreats, and conferences. Together, they founded Heartstream Resources, Inc.

Dr. Dodds earned three graduate degrees, in developmental psychology, in education, and in organizational systems, including a doctorate at UCSB. She holds two counseling licenses and has more than twenty thousand hours of practice. She is the author of more than a dozen books and over one hundred published articles. She lectures frequently at international conferences related to mental health and humanitarian work.

Visit the website at www.heartstreamresources.org, or email at heartstreamresources@hotmail.com.

References

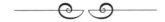

Fleming, N. D., and C. Mills. 1992. "Not Another Inventory, Rather a Catalyst for Reflection." *To Improve the Academy* 11: 137–155. https://vark-learn.com/wp-content/uploads/2014/08/not_another_inventory.pdf.

Greenberg, Melanie, PhD. March 30, 2016. "The Science of Love and Attachment: How understanding your brain chemicals can help you build lasting love." *Psychology Today.* https://www.psychologytoday.com/us/blog/the-mindful-self-express/201603/the-science-love-and-attachment.

Mayo Clinic staff. Nov. 13, 2020. "Forgiveness: Letting Go of Grudges and Bitterness." *Healthy Lifestyle: Adult Health.* www.mayoclinic.org/healthy-lifestyles/adult-health/in-depth/forgiveness/art-20047692.

Merriam-Webster.com Dictionary, s.v. "forgiveness." Accessed April 15, 2020. https://www.merriam-webster.com/dictionary/forgiveness.

Tsur, Michal. 2014. "Research Confirms Video Improves Learning Results." Accessed March 24, 2020. *Huffpost.* https://www.huffpost.com/entry/research-confirms-video-i_b_5064181.

Scripture References

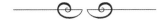

Free Online, Zondervan (NIV). https://www.coursef.com/free-online-zondervan-study-bible.

Chapter 5

Matthew 6:12 (NIV)
Proverbs 12:25 (NIV)

Chapter 6

Mark 10:8 (NIV)

Chapter 7

Proverbs 3:13–18 (NIV)

Free Online, https://www.kingjamesbibleonline.org.

Chapter 10

John 3:16 (KJV)
Jeremiah 29:12,13 (KJV)
John 8:32 (KJV)
Ephesians 1:18–19 (NIV)
1 Peter 2:29 (KJV)
Romans 3:23 (KJV)
Philippians 2:9–11 (KJV)
Romans 10:9 (KJV)
Numbers 6:24–26 (KJV)

Response/Evaluation Sheet

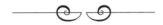

If you have used this book as a therapeutic tool with clients or used the IA prints as a personal healing guide, the author is interested in your thoughts and qualitative results.

Please complete the following questions and mail to Karen Erdman, 2259 E. Main St., Sacramento, Pennsylvania 17968.

Author contact information: kerdman@hotmail.com

1. Name of therapist or self

   _____

2. Contact information

   _____

   _____

3. Name of private practice, organization, if applicable

   _____

   _____

4. Initials of client(s), if applicable

   _____

5. Gender of client(s), or self

   _____

6. Which interactive print did you use?

   _____

7. Was the print useful? If so, in what way?

   _____

   _____

   _____

8. How did the client (or you) respond?

_____

_____

9. What are your overall impressions of using the IA prints?

_____

_____

_____

_____

Comments/suggestions

_____

_____

_____

_____

Signature or initials of therapist or self

_____

By providing your signature or initials, you are giving permission for the above information to be used in advertising or for research purposes.

Notes:

Notes:

Notes:

Printed in the United States
by Baker & Taylor Publisher Services